YOUR KNOWLEDGE HAS VALUE

- We will publish your bachelor's and
  master's thesis, essays and papers

- Your own eBook and book -
  sold worldwide in all relevant shops

- Earn money with each sale

Upload your text at www.GRIN.com
and publish for free

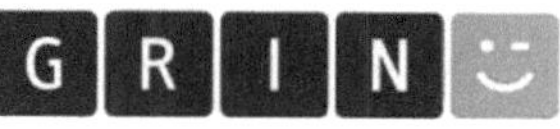

Tushar Chatterji

Metabolomic responses to Recombinant Human Erythropoietin administration

GRIN Verlag

Bibliografische Information der Deutschen Nationalbibliothek:

Die Deutsche Bibliothek verzeichnet diese Publikation in der Deutschen National-
bibliografie; detaillierte bibliografische Daten sind im Internet über http://dnb.d-
nb.de/ abrufbar.

Imprint:

Copyright © 2011 GRIN Verlag GmbH
Druck und Bindung: Books on Demand GmbH, Norderstedt Germany
ISBN: 978-3-656-13865-5

Metabolomic responses to Recombinant Human Erythropoietin administration

Tushar Chatterji

College of Medical, Veterinary and Life Sciences

University of Glasgow

March 2011

Abstract

Metabolomics is the comprehensive analysis of the metabolite profiles within a biological system. r-HuEPO stimulates red blood cell production, thereby enhancing maximal oxygen delivery to the tissues. The ergogenic potential of r-HuEPO, demonstrated through improved aerobic capacity and performance has reported r-HuEPO to be the most widely abused erythropoietic stimulant till date. This study was aimed at determining the effects of r-HuEPO on the human metabolome by analyzing metabolites from blood plasma and urine. Analysis of these metabolites was then used to determine how such metabolic interactions affected physiological status and exercise performance. Three well trained individuals participated in the study. Blood and urine were collected from the subjects. Plasma and urine samples were analyzed for metabolites by LC-MS Orbitrap and data was analyzed in the form of heatmaps and PCA plots. Further data interpretations for metabolites of interest were performed by a software, mzMatch/PeakML. Analysis of the human metabolome revealed 1000 metabolites which were manually categorized into 190 human metabolites. Significant metabolite patterns in response to r-HuEPO suggested the physiological effects of r-HuEPO on certain metabolites. A better understanding of the metabolic changes mediated by r-HuEPO might provide an insight into the metabolic signals in response to exercise performance.

Abbreviations

EPO- Erythropoietin

r-HuEPO- Recombinant Human Erythropoietin

MS- Mass Spectrometry

LC-MS- Liquid Chromatography-Mass Spectrometry

NMR- Nuclear Magnetic Resonance

GC-TOF/MS- Gas Chromatography-Time of Flight/Mass Spectrometry

EPS- Erythropoietic Stimulant

ETT- Exercise Treadmill Test

WADA- World Anti-Doping Agency

PCA- Perchloric Acid

HMDB- Human Metabolite Database

KEGG- Kyoto Encyclopaedia of Genes and Genomes

NEG- Negative Ionization Mode

RSD- Relative Standard Deviation

PCA- Principal Component Analysis

PC(s)-Principal Component(s)

ACN- Acetonitrile

Introduction

Metabolomics, a part of 'OMICS' sciences, is the identification and quantification of all metabolites (lipids, vitamins, small peptides and protein co-factors) in a biological system [33, 38]. Metabolomics is progressing as an important tool in systems biology in combination with genomics, transcriptomics and proteomics [2, 4] (figure 1). In relation to exercise physiology, metabolomics focuses on metabolite-rich body fluids such as blood plasma and urine [18, 33]. Plasma plays a crucial role in metabolite transportation throughout the body while urine samples are easy to collect for metabolomics analysis [3, 10]. Since metabolites are difficult to analyze in a single analysis they could be grouped into specific classes, analyzed and data restored electronically to provide necessary qualitative and quantitative information [15]. MS and NMR are the main technologies used in metabolomic studies [10, 33]. Based on the nature of metabolites, LC-MS Orbitrap was used for metabolite analysis due to high chromatographic resolution, sensitivity and superior quantitative analysis [22, 23]. EPO is a hormone produced primarily by the kidneys [11, 13]. EPO is the key regulator of RBC formation by stimulating differentiation of erythroid progenitor cells, a process known as erythropoiesis [11, 13]. r-HuEPO, a genetically modified form of EPO, has been found to significantly improve aerobic performance in athletes by accelerating RBC production and enhancing maximal oxygen delivery to the tissues [1, 13, 37].

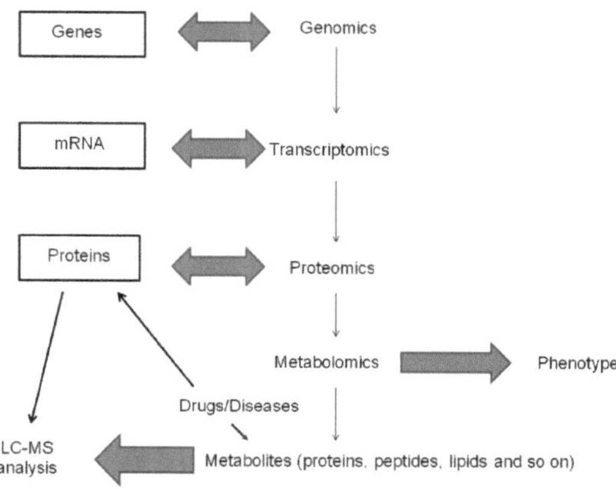

Figure 1. Outline of the 'OMICS' cascade: The diagram represents the stages from genes to metabolites which are eventually analyzed by LC-MS. The relay of genetic information to subsequent higher levels is demonstrated. Differences in the metabolite levels may reflect their corresponding enzymatic activities. Metabolite profiles may also be altered by changes in drug concentrations or kinetics (pharmacokinetics) and/or by disease onset or progression. In association with the other 'OMICS' technologies, metabolomics aims to combine data and provide useful information on the physiological status of an individual (i.e. the phenotype) [33, 45].

In conjunction with exercise, metabolic interactions can be assessed on the basis of complex nutrients in combination with advanced multivariate statistics and interpretation tools [7, 15, 47]. In a study performed on professional athletes subjected to strength-endurance training (i.e. rowing), metabolomic differences between rowers and control subjects with prolonged training was determined by monitoring the level of endogenous metabolites by GC-TOF/MS during the training program [47]. The study demonstrated how metabolites such as alanine, lactate, cysteine, glutamic acid, free fatty acids, pyroglutamic acid, tyrosine and glutamine affected glucose and energy metabolism, oxidative stress, lipolysis and amino acid metabolism, thus providing an understanding of the rowers' physiological status during intensive exercise [47].

Another study demonstrated the comprehensive metabolic profiling of the human plasma suggesting significant changes in twenty-three metabolites in the plasma at peak exercise [26]. Up-regulation in the glycolytic and lipolytic pathways, amino acids and purine catabolism was observed and these results were in conjunction with rises in lactate, pyruvate, glycerol, alanine and glutamine and a reduction in acetoacetate respectively [20, 26]. Increased levels of 3-phosphoglyceric acid and glucose-6 phosphate in plasma were also observed after an ETT [26]. Plasma metabolic profiles of fumarate, malate and succinate were individually affected in the tri-carboxylic acid cycle by exercise while α-ketoglutarate remained unchanged [8, 16, 32]. In concordance with such interesting findings from the human metabolome, the aim of this study was to investigate the complex interactions between multiple metabolites obtained from plasma and urine in the human metabolome and determine how these metabolites get affected by r-HuEPO administration. A careful analysis of these metabolites would further help interpret the physiological status of athletes, prevent misuse of r-HuEPO and determine alternative strategies to doping detection [8].

Design and Methods

Subjects

The study involved three well trained individuals (**mean ± SD**, age: 25.7 ± 5.7 years, weight: 69.7 ± 2.3 kg, height: 177.3 ± 1.7 cm). All subjects were university students and were allowed to continue their respective training sessions and maintain a healthy lifestyle throughout the study period. However, none of the subjects participated in a competition during the course of the study [43]. The subjects underwent an initial medical examination a week before the study commenced. The study was conducted according to the World Medical Association (**Declaration of Helsinki**) and was reviewed and approved by WADA and the Glasgow University Ethics Committee. All subjects were informed of the duration, experimental procedures and risks involved in the study and were included after having given their written consent [19, 35, 43].

Study design

The trial was divided into three phases: pre-treatment, treatment with r-HuEPO, and post-treatment/wash-out phase. The experimental protocol lasted 10 weeks with two weeks for baseline and four weeks each for r-HuEPO treatment and wash-out phases (figure 2). Following initial testing, blood and urine samples were collected from the subjects twice during baseline for metabolomics (figure 2). During the r-HuEPO administration phase, the subjects received subcutaneous injections of r-HuEPO (Epoietin beta, NeoRecormon®, Roche, Welwyn Garden City, UK) every two days for a period of 4 weeks (i.e. a total of 15 injections in 4 weeks) at a dose of 50 IU/kg body mass [35]. Iron was administered orally in the form of a 200 mg ferrous sulphate tablet (Almus Pharmaceuticals, Actavis, Barnstaple, UK) for haem synthesis [19, 43]. Blood and urine was collected thrice during this phase (figure 2). The post-treatment phase was focused on demonstrating the effects of r-HuEPO on the metabolic status of the subject, based on which the physiological conditions of the subjects were also determined. There were three sampling points for blood and urine (figure 2). This phase alleviated r-HuEPO concentrations gradually from the circulatory system of the subjects allowing them to participate in future competitions without the risk of being caught.

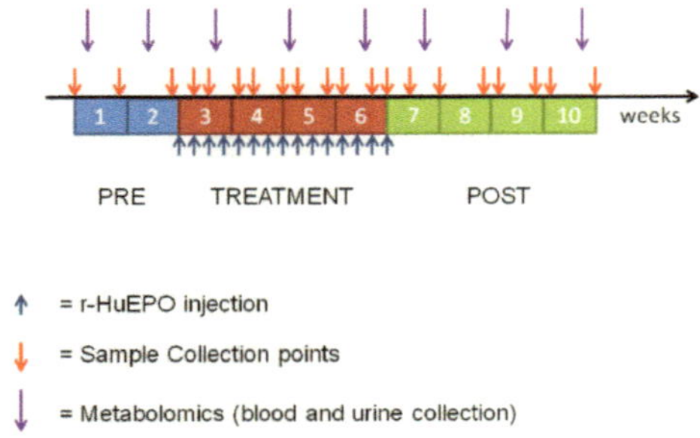

Figure 2.10 weeks trial protocol of the r-HuEPO study: The diagram not only shows the sample collection points (total of 20, red arrows) for all subjects throughout the study, but also the sampling points for blood and urine collection for metabolomics during the three phases (i.e. Baseline/pre-treatment:(2), treatment with r-HuEPO:(3) and post-treatment:(3)) represented by purple arrows. The time points at which r-HuEPO was administered to the subjects during the treatment phase is also indicated by thick blue arrows.

Blood/Urine collection

Phlebotomy was performed either by canulation or venipuncture depending upon the experimental tests the subjects underwent on that particular visit. Each blood sample was collected into a 4 ml K$_2$EDTA tube (Vacuette®, Greiner bio-one, Austria), a 3.5 ml serum tube (Vacutainer, BD, Belliver Industrial Estate, Plymouth, UK) and a 5 ml clear tube (Sterilin, UK) from an anticubital vein before the trial protocol-twice during baseline, thrice during the acceleration and wash-out phases. The subject was asked to lie down facing up (supine position) for venipuncture [43]. Following blood collection, 1 ml of plasma from the EDTA-vacutainer-system was extracted after centrifugation at 4000 g for 15 minutes on a bench top centrifuge (Universal 320R, Zentrifugen, Germany) into a 1.8 ml cryotube (Alpha Laboratories, Eastleigh, Hampshire, UK), placed in a cryobox and stored at -80°C (figure 3). Urine samples collected from the subjects in a 20 ml clear tube was divided into three aliquots of 1 ml each in1.8 ml cryotubes, placed in the cryobox and stored at -80°C (figure 3). Urine aliquots were prepared immediately after their collection and stored at -80°C to inhibit metabolic reactions completely before proceeding to collect plasma samples. The protocol for blood collection also involved addition of 2.5% (0.3 N) PCA to blood in the EDTA-vacutainer-system (figure 3).

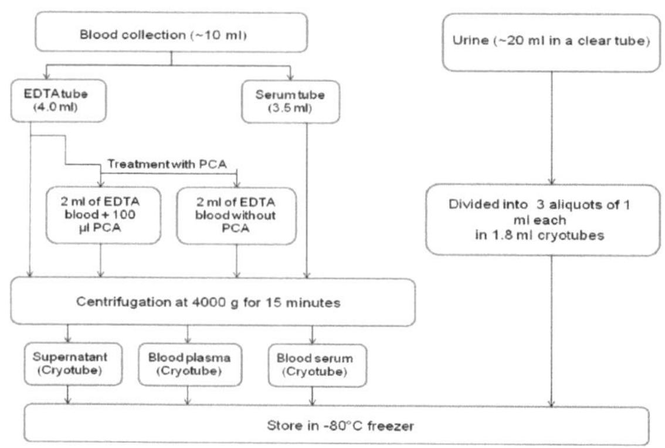

Figure 3. Protocol for sample collection for metabolomics: Blood plasma and urine were extracted from the subjects for metabolite analysis. Perchloric Acid, abbreviated as PCA was used as a deproteinization agent to inhibit the metabolic reactions immediately after blood collection in the EDTA tube. A modified protocol (see discussion) involved replacing PCA with HPLC-grade Acetonitrile (ACN) in the ratio of 3:1 (3 ml of ACN:1 ml of whole blood). The plasma and urine samples were stored at -80°C for further analysis by LC-MS.

Sample analysis by LC-MS and Statistical interpretation

Blood plasma and urine samples were transferred to the University of Strathclyde mass spectrometry laboratory for metabolite analysis by LC-MS (Exactive Orbitrap, Thermo Fisher Scientific). Orbitrap maintains steady performance levels by accurately measuring masses quickly making it congruous with chromatography [22, 46]. Sample concentrations < 1 ng/ml and ranges approximating 10^5 can be reached by the Orbitrap [30]. Once raw data is obtained from LC-MS, metabolites of biological interest are characterized by databases. The databases used in this study were HMDB (http://www.hmdb.ca/) and the KEGG database (http://www.genome.jp/kegg/ligand.html) [45]. Following characterization, PCA was used to process the LC-MS data. PCA is a multivariate statistical technique which breaks down highly correlated variables into smaller uncorrelated variables called PCs [28]. This provides the systematic data variation in the original sample pool [7]. It identifies the most important gradients in the data ensuring maximum variability. Each PC was linearly related to the original data points and orthogonally limited, thus independent of any other PCs [7, 47]. This reduces data dimensionality from LC-MS data and retrieves maximum information. The outcomes of the PCA were obtained in the form of score plots. The scatter diagram of the plots along two axes (PC1 and PC2) differentiated identical metabolites which were clustered together from unrelated metabolites located further away [47]. mzMatch/PeakML is a data processing software used for analyzing LC-MS data for metabolomics written in a computer language, Java. This tool simplified the processing steps in LC-MS data analysis (http://mzmatch.sourceforge.net/).

Results

Metabolic profiling of blood plasma and urine was performed for all three subjects and cross-referenced with mzMatch/PeakML software (for subject 1) to identify metabolites of interest. A total of 1000 metabolite peaks were obtained from the mass chromatogram. An analysis of these peaks manually identified approximately 367, 233 and 178 metabolites corresponding to the three subjects respectively. These metabolites were then categorized into human, non-human, xenobiotics and unknown after matching them with HMDB and KEGG databases.

Subject 1

Manual interpretation

Of 367 metabolite peaks, around 192 human metabolites were identified for this subject. The data was then analysed by means of heatmaps and PCA plots. The heatmaps obtained from blood plasma and urine showed all identified background ions (figure 4). The most variable metabolite peaks were identified according to the intensity of the signals from the LC-MS data. The heatmap for plasma suggested changes in the metabolite patterns in the post treatment phase as the intensity of the colour varied. In other terms, the yellow colour observed on the maps was indicative of these metabolites getting down-regulated (figure 4). The metabolite pattern did not significantly change from baseline to treatment (as suggested by the colour intensity remaining orange in figure 4). It was difficult to conclude whether this was due to r-HuEPO effects or contamination during the sampling and/or data processing stages.

The heatmap for urine showed variations in the data set for all phases. Certain metabolites observed in the post phase were comparable to baseline with very little variation during the treatment phase. This meant that some of the metabolites might be correlated (figure 4). The relatively small change observed during the treatment phase indicated that r-HuEPO did not have a significant effect on the metabolites. Some major patterns were consistently visible from the PCA plots for plasma and urine because the plots for the post phase were present in a different cluster far away from baseline and treatment (figure 5). This pattern was not only visible when the metabolite data was "logged" to reduce the influence of extreme values on the results, but also when the most variable peaks were considered at a RSD>1 (figure 5C). The close clustering of baseline and treatment plots was indicative of an unchanged metabolite pattern. On the other hand, the PCA plots from urine deviated drastically from the desired trend in the data pool. The score plots were clustered around the same area making identification of the three phases difficult (figure 6A,6C). This meant that the plots calculated from the three phases were in the same gradient and maximum variability in data between the two axes (PC1 and PC2 respectively) was not visible. Metabolite identification would be difficult, even if some of the metabolites were actually affected r-HuEPO.

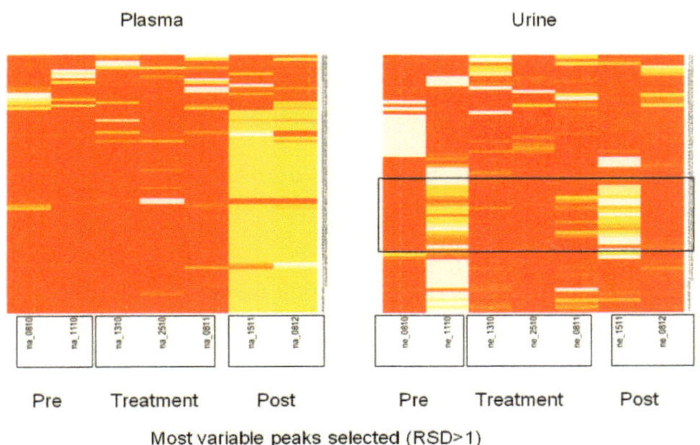

Figure 4. Heatmap for plasma and urine from subject 1: The heatmap represented the data from LC-MS. The x and y axes (unmarked) represented retention time and mass/charge ratio

respectively. Specific metabolite patterns were identified from the vast majority of background ions. The intensity of the signal corresponded to the colour on the heatmap. The plasma heatmap on the left showed a significant up-regulation of metabolites post-rHuEPO and no variation in pattern during baseline and r-HuEPO phases. The urine heatmap on the right revealed better metabolite patterns with up-regulation observed in the post phase of certain metabolites (highlighted region).

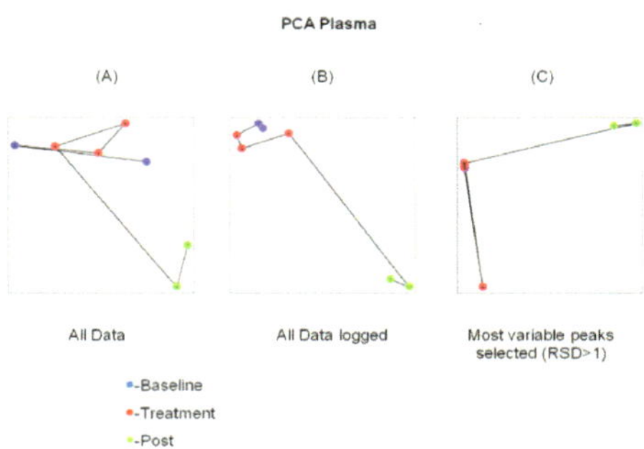

Figure 5.PCA plots from the plasma for subject 1: Principal Component Analysis, abbreviated as PCA represented a simplified form of the data variation in the original metabolite pool. The x-axis and y-axis (unmarked) represented the first and second principal component respectively. (A) The plot represented the complete metabolite dataset. (B) The "logged data" was obtained by considering the logarithm of LC-MS data. (C) The most variable peaks were selected and plotted at a RSD>1. The three phases have been separated by numbers and colours (1 and 2, blue for baseline, 3, 4 and 5, red for treatment and 6 and 7, green for post treatment). Note the variation in the data pattern for all plots and the characteristic separation of the post phase from baseline and r-HuEPO treatment phases.

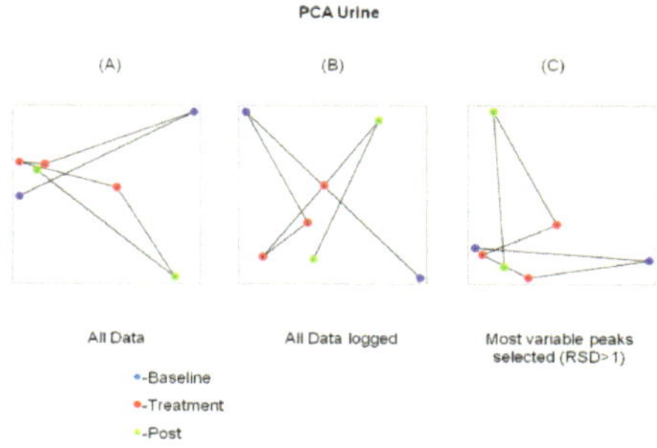

Interpretation via mzMatch/PeakML

The metabolite data for this subject was also interpreted via the software tool mzMatch/PeakML. The heatmap and PCA plots for plasma metabolites were obtained in NEG. This mode of ionization mainly detected phosphates and organic acids which formed a part of the tricarboxylic acid cycle (63). 318 metabolite peaks were identified in the heatmap. When the most variable peaks were investigated at a RSD>0.5, an interesting pattern was observed in a portion of the heatmap (highlighted region of figure 7). The metabolites in this region were down-regulated in the treatment phase while maintaining an almost identical metabolite pattern in the post phase when compared to the pre-treatment phase. This might mean that r-HuEPO provided a stimulatory effect on selected metabolites to the extent of making it comparable to baseline metabolite levels. However, r-HuEPO was down-regulated in the patterns for these metabolites (figure 7). Further analysis of the metabolites in this region and their corresponding roles in the biochemical/metabolic pathways might relate the actions of r-HuEPO on metabolic status.

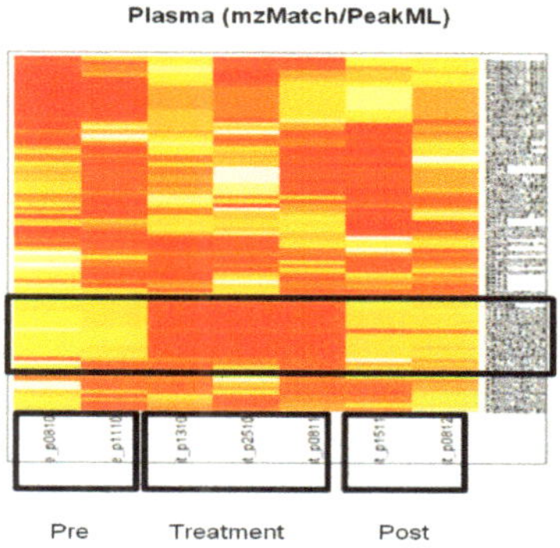

Plasma (mzMatch/PeakML)

Pre   Treatment   Post

Figure 7. Heatmap for plasma via mzMatch/PeakML for subject 1: Heatmap was generated in the same way as manual interpretation. The x and y axes represented retention time and mass over charge ratio respectively. A strong correlation was found between the metabolites in the pre and post phases (highlighted region). Note that the variation in intensity possibly because of the contaminants in the list of most variable signals.

The PCA plots from plasma were also obtained in NEG. As seen in the heatmap, the PCA plots detected 318 metabolite peaks (figure 8). This was comparable to the PCA analysis obtained manually as data clustering in the post phase was located far away from baseline and treatment score plots (figure 5). The results suggested an increase in the level of endogenous metabolites from the treatment to the post phase. Further analysis could confirm whether this rise was due to a "real" effect caused by r-HuEPO or machine drift. This would depend on the order in which the samples were analysed by LC-MS. Lactate was extracted in NEG via mzMatch/PeakML after individual metabolites were serially identified. An increasing trend in lactate was observed which corresponded to a fold change of approximately 1.3 (figure 9). These results correlated to the trend observed for lactate from raw data suggesting that r-HuEPO might have had an effect on lactate influx post administration. The shapes of the peaks detected via the software were also good having an accuracy of <1 ppm indicative of high data acquisition quality (figure 10).

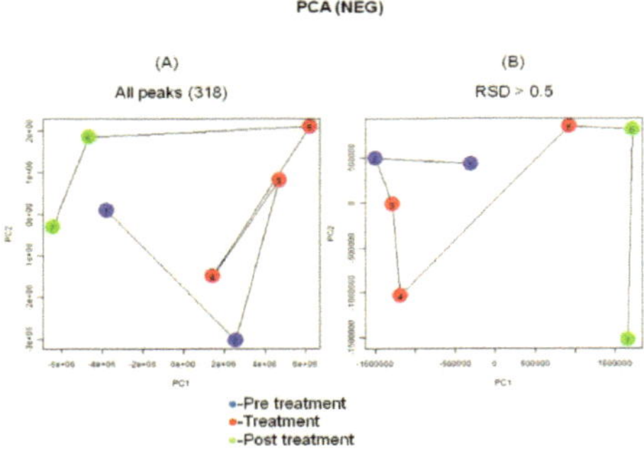

Figure 8.PCA plots for plasma via mzMatch/PeakML of subject 1: The score plots were obtained in negative ionization mode (NEG). (A) The metabolite peaks corresponding to 318 metabolites were plotted. (B) The most variable metabolic signals were obtained at a RSD>0.5. Note the variation in data from baseline to post r-HuEPO phase.

Subject 2

Around 233 metabolites were identified. The data was interpreted in the same way as subject 1. The data from the plasma heatmap showed significant changes in the metabolite patterns in the lower region of the heatmap (figure 10). These metabolites were gradually affected by r-HuEPO in the treatment phase. An up-regulation in these metabolites was observed in the post phase. Other regions of the heatmap showed little evidence of the patterns that were expected. The heatmap for urine, with the exception of a few patterns, showed an increase in the metabolite clusters in the post phase (middle region of figure 10). Like in the case of plasma, few metabolites seemed to be up-regulated by r-HuEPO but this might not necessarily be affected by r-HuEPO. Despite observing a shift in the "logged" data for PCA analysis in plasma and urine, there was no variability in the metabolite patterns in both cases as data clustering for all phases occurred in the same region of the plot. Significant changes in the metabolite patterns could not be predicted through the different phases (figure11, 12).

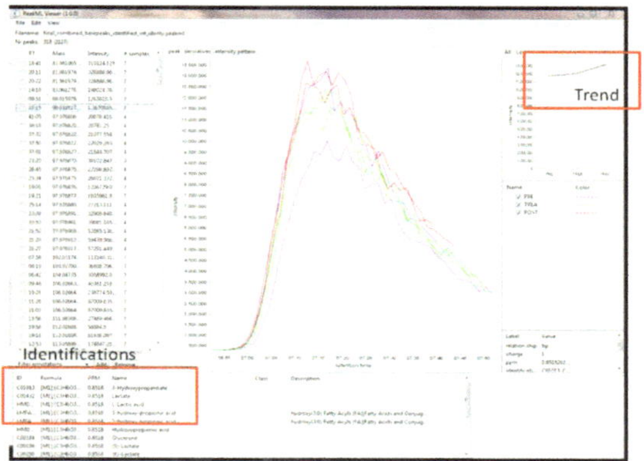

Figure 9. Peak extracted for plasma lactate via mzMatch/PeakML for subject 1: The figure demonstrates the typical pattern in which metabolite peaks are identified by mzMatch/PeakML. The peaks were obtained in the negative ionization mode. The data showed an increasing trend (~1.3 fold change) from treatment to the post phase (upper right corner). The peak quality was good and reproducible with an accuracy of <1 ppm. Note the changes in colour distinguishing the three phases (purple for baseline, green for treatment and red for post).

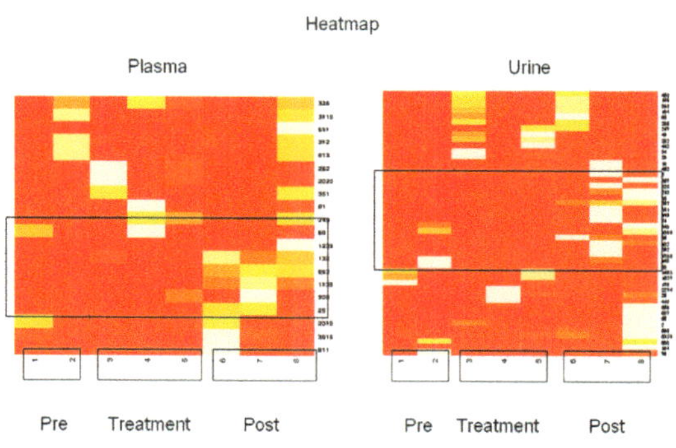

Figure 10. Heatmap for plasma and urine of subject 2: The heatmap identified metabolites of interest against the background ions. The plasma heatmap (left) showed a change in the intensity of certain metabolites in the post phase (highlighted area). No change was observed under r-HuEPO effects. The urine heatmap (right) complied with plasma as up-regulation was observed after r-HuEPO administration.

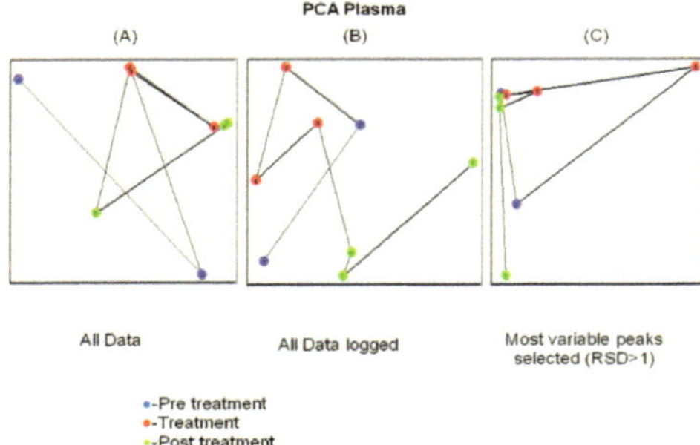

Figure 11.PCA plots from the blood plasma of subject 2: The x and y axes (unmarked) represent the first and second principal components respectively. (A) The scatter diagram in the form of score plots distinguished metabolites in the three phases from the entire metabolite data pool. (B) The data was "logged" to reduce the effect of extreme values on the plots. (C) The most variable metabolic signals were plotted at a RSD>1. Note the distinct variation in data for the post phases in figure (B).

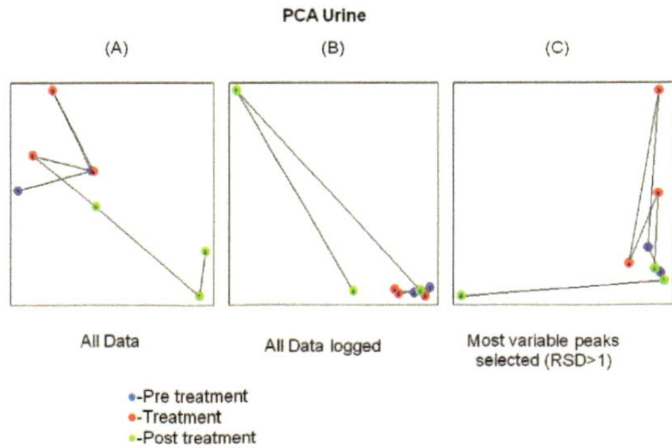

Figure 12.PCA plots from urine of subject 2: The x and y axes (not shown) represented PC1 and PC2 respectively. (A) The score plot comprising complete metabolite data was obtained. (B) The logarithmic values of the peaks were calculated and plotted to minimise the effects of extreme values. (C) The most variable peaks were plotted at a RSD>1. The plots for the three phases were differentiated by their respective colours and numbers (1 & 2, blue-pre treatment, 3, 4 & 5, red-treatment, 6, 7 & 8, green-post treatment). Note the characteristic separation of the post phase from baseline and treatment in (A) and (B).

Subject 3

Around 178 metabolites were identified by LC-MS. Although some metabolites were correlated in the baseline phase of the heatmap for plasma (lower region of figure 13), a significant trend in metabolite patterns was not observed possibly because r-HuEPO down-regulated these metabolites during the administration phase (figure 13). The heatmap for urine demonstrated that certain metabolites were up-regulated during the treatment phase and they continued to maintain an identical metabolite pattern in the post treatment phase (figure 13). However, the PCA plots for plasma did not provide any data corresponding to r-HuEPO effects as data points for all phases were clustered closely. It was difficult to determine if any major metabolites were affected by r-HuEPO either in the administration or post treatment phases (figure 14). A similar pattern was observed in urine PCA plots. The presence of endogenous metabolites in the same cluster prevented the maximum variability that would be expected in the metabolite patterns (figure 15).

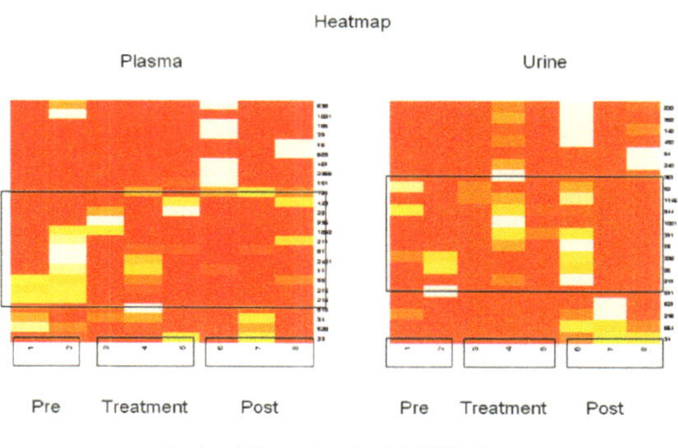

Figure 13. Heatmap representation for plasma and urine from subject 3: The heatmap represented the LC-MS data and identified metabolites against background ions. Significant changes in metabolite patterns were observed in baseline samples for certain metabolites in the plasma (left) and urine (right) heatmaps. Some of the patterns were affected during r-HuEPO treatment (highlighted area). A down-regulation was observed in the same metabolites in the post phase.

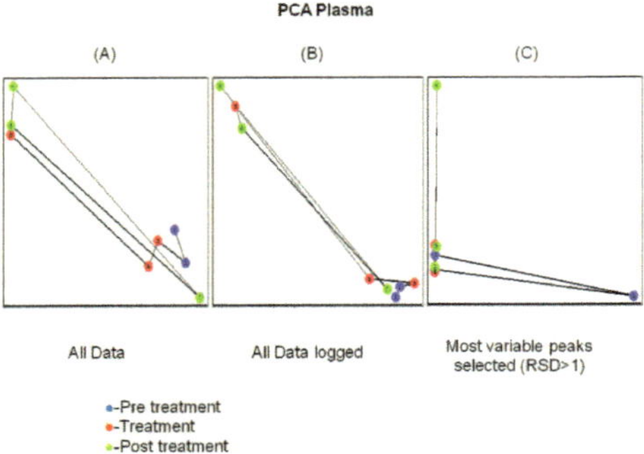

Figure 14.PCA plots of blood plasma from subject 3: The clustering of the data on the two axes (PC1 and PC2) (not shown) represented the metabolite patterns obtained from the three phases of the subject. (A) The score plots comprising the entire metabolite dataset. (B) The data was "logged" to reduce the effect of the maximum values on peaks of interest. (C) The variable metabolite peaks were separated at a RSD>1. Note metabolites were located in the same gradient of the plots for all phases (marked in respective colours and numbers).

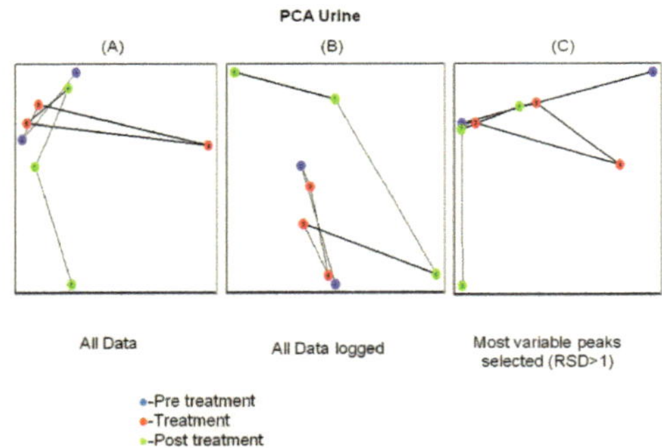

Figure 15.PCA plots for urine from subject 3: (A) The data represented the complete metabolite data set from LC-MS analysis. (B) The plots were obtained after considering the logarithm of the peaks to minimise the effects of extreme values on scores. (C) The most variable peaks were plotted at a RSD>1. The phases were classified by their respective colours and numbers (1 and 2, blue for baseline, 3, 4 and 5, red for treatment, 6, 7 and 8, green for post r-HuEPO). Note the desired variation between the three phases in (B).

Comparisons of lactate influx during baseline, treatment and post phases into the metabolic system of the three subjects demonstrated the physiological and biological effects of r-

HuEPO on lactate exchange [8] . The subjects achieved higher lactate levels in the post phase when compared to baseline and r-HuEPO phases (figure 16). Lactate which was maintained at a stable range during baseline and treatment showed an increasing trend in the post phase for subject 1. A similar pattern was observed for subjects 2 and 3 in the post phase but with lower lactate levels. A down-regulation observed in the treatment phase of subject 3 suggested that r-HuEPO might have an inhibitory effect on lactate during administration (figure 16). The results demonstrated the potential of r-HuEPO to enhance lactate uptake possibly via a hydrogen ion carrier protein, MCT-1, thus establishing lactate as a vital mediator of metabolism [5, 8].

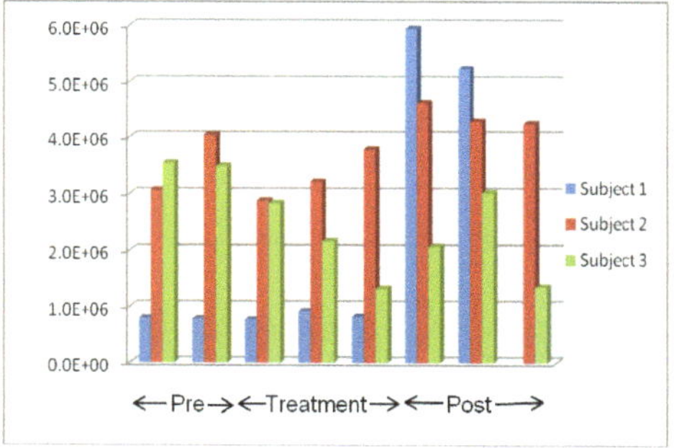

Figure 16. Lactate levels from all three subjects for all phases: The diagram summarized the changes observed in lactate levels from baseline till post-rHuEPO. The x and y axes represented the three phases of the study and semi-quantitative MS data readings (arbitrary units) respectively. Subject 1 achieved the highest lactate influx (as seen in post phase). Subjects 2 and 3 also experienced a rise in lactate levels during post phase. Note the decline in lactate during r-HuEPO phase for subject 3.

Discussion

Metabolic profiling of blood plasma and urine provided a comprehensive analysis of the human metabolome [26]. Metabolites of interest were characterized using LC-MS and distinct patterns were deciphered using heatmaps and PCA plots. Despite many variations in the metabolite data, the heatmaps for plasma and urine provided some significant metabolite patterns for all subjects. Certain major patterns were also consistently visible from the PCA plots of plasma and urine. Some samples were characterized by increased levels of correlated metabolites but not necessarily the ones which would be expected to be affected by r-HuEPO. A rise in pyruvate, glycerol, alanine and glutamine levels and a decline in acetoacetate concentration in response to r-HuEPO administration are suitable predictions if the metabolome is further investigated with the help of sophisticated software tools [20, 26]. The use of such software technologies might enhance data processing and accuracy by detecting significant trends and fold changes in some major metabolite patterns.

Some important metabolites resulting from plasma metabolic variations such as niacinamide, a mediator of insulin release and allantoin (a product of uric acid), a key regulator of oxidative stress might be expected to show significant up-regulation and down-regulation respectively if properly identified and quantified [9, 21, 26, 36]. However, such metabolites sometimes go undetected as their concentrations remain too low in the metabolome. High signal-to-noise ratio in certain parts of the heatmap may further undermine the detection of certain critical metabolites. The enormous clustering of data and "logged" data centred around the same point in some score plots prevented maximum variability and reduction in data dimensionality. This is why PCA should be assisted with supervised methodologies such as OPLS and OPLS-DA to improve data structure and analysis [28, 45]. On the other hand, changes in the plasma metabolite concentrations cause significant fold changes in some of the components of the TCA cycle, namely fumarate, malate and succinate [16, 27]. It would be interesting to conduct future experiments to determine the effects of r-HuEPO on these constituents and correlate the observed changes to exercise performance and fitness of athletes [26]. The difficulties in data interpretation could also be attributed to the lack of technical replicates (i.e. fewer sampling points during sample collection) because analysis, prediction and comparison of metabolite patterns and their relevance in the metabolic pathways would technically become easier with duplicate and/or triplicate entities.

After serially identifying all the metabolites within the human metabolome, lactate was characterized both manually and by the mzMatch/PeakML software. This was in concordance with studies demonstrating the potential of r-HuEPO to significantly affect lactate influx via a hydrogen ion protein carrier, MCT-1 [8, 25, 31]. The present study showed increased levels of lactate post r-HuEPO administration in the three subjects suggesting that r-HuEPO might have caused up-regulation in lactate levels in plasma. Analysis via the software tool further indicated an increasing trend and a fold change of approximately 1.3, thus demonstrating the role of r-HuEPO in modifying lactate metabolism at rest [6, 8, 32]. However, in order to completely justify the role of r-HuEPO in lactate exchange, further studies need to be performed to calculate lactate kinetics which might not only provide a better explanation for lactate metabolism either at rest or during exercise, but also suggest why individuals placed (as seen in the post phase of subject 1) [5, 8].

Metabolomics is a complex approach since metabolites are affected by even the slightest variations, either analytical or biological [39]. These variations might occur at any stage of the metabolomics strategy (figure 17). So, care should be taken from the sampling stage. Blood and urine samples were collected from the subjects in resting phase. Fasting samples (homeostatic) provide less information in metabolomics analysis [18, 29, 41]. This might partly explain the variation in the data from the PCA plots of plasma and urine. Since plasma and urine possess specific biological characteristics, sampling, sample collection and storage must be addressed [29, 44]. In order to minimise diurnal variations, urine samples were collected from the subjects immediately after their arrival in the laboratory [29]. The use of a suitable anticoagulant is also important while collecting plasma samples to reduce the possibilities of unwanted peaks during chromatogram analysis [39]. For this reason, an EDTA-vacutainer system was used for plasma collection [14]. Selecting an appropriate deproteinization agent for plasma is a critical step during sample collection in metabolomics [10]. Treatment of whole blood with perchloric acid proved to be disadvantageous as it masked the peaks corresponding to some major metabolites in the chromatographic analysis (data not shown). It was replaced with HPLC-grade ACN, which resulted in the quantification of more low molecular weight metabolites and a suitable signal-to-noise ratio for analysis [10].

Limitations

Metabolomics is faced with a lot of challenges [17, 24]. The range of low molecular weight metabolites that make up the metabolome presents a challenge with regards to their analysis, identification and biological interpretation [4, 12, 24]. Quantitative analysis at the level of the individual metabolites should be investigated to provide a better understanding of the biochemical pathways [12, 15, 17]. Justifiable modifications need to be made to simplify the huge volumes of data that is obtained from the metabolite pool [39]. This problem might be resolved by developing a database identical to GenBank or PDB which will help generate a common reference spectra to identify metabolites of interest, thereby improving the reliability and validity of the metabolomics data [39, 42]. With respect to technology, LC-MS poses disadvantages such as ion suppression [40, 46]. This is caused when the background ions compete with ions of interest for space within the Orbitrap analyzer under the influence of

environmental stresses [22, 23]. Although Orbitrap can achieve dynamic ranges as high as

10^5, it does not provide extensive metabolite coverage due to space-charge constraints within

the ion trap [30, 46].

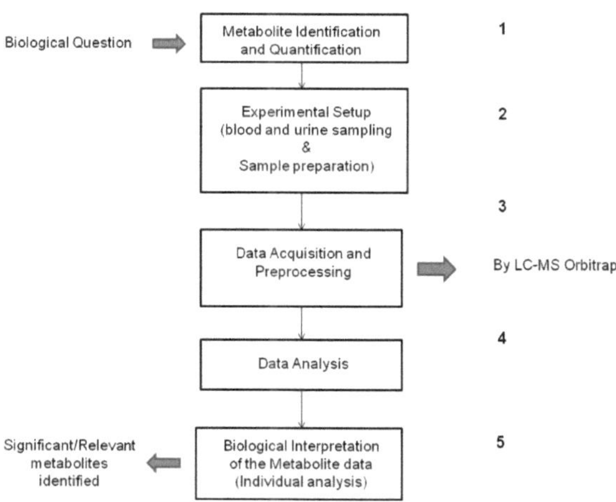

Figure 17. Flowchart of the metabolomics strategy: The diagram shows the steps beginning from the identification of metabolites up to the interpretation of the biological question by quantifying metabolites which play a significant role in the human metabolome. (1) The aim would always be to identify those metabolites which significantly affect the human metabolome (in this study, the impact that r-HuEPO had on these metabolites). (2) The experimental design involving blood and urine sampling, collection and storage for further analysis. (3) Once samples have been prepared for analysis, high-performance acquisition and pre-processing methods are used to obtain the best LC-MS profiles after matching all metabolite profiles to the reference database. The instrument used in this study was the LC-MS Orbitrap. (4) The data obtained from the profiles were analyzed with the help of software tools which presented the data in a readable text format (".txt"). (5) The final stage involved interpretation of the data and the identification of relevant metabolites in the human metabolome followed by a careful investigation into those which had a tendency to be up-regulated or down-regulated by r-HuEPO [2, 22, 40, 45].

Conclusion

Fraught with challenges and obstacles in almost every stage of the metabolomics approach, this branch of 'OMICS cascade' still keeps the hopes of researchers alive who aim to integrate this field with genomics, proteomics and transcriptomics and create a revolution in the field of scientific research [2, 33, 38]. In the words of Mitchell *et al.* "Occasionally, a new idea emerges that has the potential to revolutionize the entire field of scientific endeavour. It is now within our grasp to be able to detect subtle perturbations within the phenomenally complex biochemical matrix of living organisms. The discipline of metabonomics promises an all-encompassing approach to understanding, total yet fundamental, changes occurring in disease processes, drug toxicity and cell function"[34]. In the light of this theory, a better interpretation of the metabolic changes mediated by r-HuEPO might provide an insight into the metabolic signals in response to exercise performance in athletes [8, 26, 27]. Repeated infusions of r-HuEPO might be tested to demonstrate the potential of the drug in altering substrate oxidation and lactate metabolism in athletes at rest and during exercise [5, 8]. The discovery of novel metabolites coupled with knowledge of the physiological and biological effects of r-HuEPO might help improve strategies for doping prevention and detection [8, 45].

Acknowledgement

I would like to thank my supervisor, Dr. Yannis Pitsiladis for providing me his whole-hearted guidance throughout the project. I would also like to thank PhD researchers Pantazis Takas, Jerome Durussel, and Ramzy Ross for their constant help in making this research project a success. This project would not have been possible without the valuable contributions of Liang Zheng (Scientist, Beatson Cancer Research Institute, Glasgow) and Professor Rainer Breitling (University of Glasgow) in mass spectrometry data analysis and interpretation.

References

1   Audran, M., Gareau, R., Matecki, S., Durand, F., Chenard, C., Sicart, M. T., Marion, B. and Bressolle, F. (1999) Effects of erythropoietin administration in training athletes and possible indirect detection in doping control. Medicine and science in sports and exercise. 31, 639-645

2   Bino, R. J., Hall, R. D., Fiehn, O., Kopka, J., Saito, K., Draper, J., Nikolau, B. J., Mendes, P., Roessner-Tunali, U., Beale, M. H., Trethewey, R. N., Lange, B. M., Wurtele, E. S. and Sumner, L. W. (2004) Potential of metabolomics as a functional genomics tool. Trends in plant science. 9, 418-425

3   Breidbach, A., Catlin, D. H., Green, G. A., Tregub, I., Truong, H. and Gorzek, J. (2003) Detection of recombinant human erythropoietin in urine by isoelectric focusing. Clinical chemistry. 49, 901-907

4   Breitling, R., Pitt, A. R. and Barrett, M. P. (2006) Precision mapping of the metabolome. Trends in biotechnology. 24, 543-548

5   Brooks, G. A. (1991) Current concepts in lactate exchange. Medicine and science in sports and exercise. 23, 895-906

6   Cayla, J., Lavoie, C., Gareau, R. and Duvallet, A. (1999) Effects of recombinant erythropoietin (r-HuEPO) on plasma glucose concentration in endurance-trained rats. Acta physiologica Scandinavica. 166, 247-249

7   Chorell, E., Moritz, T., Branth, S., Antti, H. and Svensson, M. B. (2009) Predictive metabolomics evaluation of nutrition-modulated metabolic stress responses in human blood

serum during the early recovery phase of strenuous physical exercise. Journal of proteome research. 8, 2966-2977

8   Connes, P., Caillaud, C., Mercier, J., Bouix, D. and Casties, J. F. (2004) Injections of recombinant human erythropoietin increases lactate influx into erythrocytes. J Appl Physiol. 97, 326-332

9   Crino, A., Schiaffini, R., Manfrini, S., Mesturino, C., Visalli, N., Beretta Anguissola, G., Suraci, C., Pitocco, D., Spera, S., Corbi, S., Matteoli, M. C., Patera, I. P., Manca Bitti, M. L., Bizzarri, C. and Pozzilli, P. (2004) A randomized trial of nicotinamide and vitamin E in children with recent onset type 1 diabetes (IMDIAB IX). European journal of endocrinology / European Federation of Endocrine Societies. 150, 719-724

10   Daykin, C. A., Foxall, P. J., Connor, S. C., Lindon, J. C. and Nicholson, J. K. (2002) The comparison of plasma deproteinization methods for the detection of low-molecular-weight metabolites by (1)H nuclear magnetic resonance spectroscopy. Analytical biochemistry. 304, 220-230

11   Delanghe, J. R., Bollen, M. and Beullens, M. (2008) Testing for recombinant erythropoietin. American journal of hematology. 83, 237-241

12   Dunn, W. B., Bailey, N. J. and Johnson, H. E. (2005) Measuring the metabolome: current analytical technologies. The Analyst. 130, 606-625

13   Elliott, S. (2008) Erythropoiesis-stimulating agents and other methods to enhance oxygen transport. British journal of pharmacology. 154, 529-541

14   Fiehn, O. and Kind, T. (2007) Metabolite profiling in blood plasma. Methods in molecular biology (Clifton, N.J. 358, 3-17

15   German, J. B., Roberts, M. A. and Watkins, S. M. (2003) Personal metabolomics as a next generation nutritional assessment. The Journal of nutrition. 133, 4260-4266

16   Gibala, M. J., MacLean, D. A., Graham, T. E. and Saltin, B. (1998) Tricarboxylic acid cycle intermediate pool size and estimated cycle flux in human muscle during exercise. The American journal of physiology. 275, E235-242

17   Gibney, M. J., Walsh, M., Brennan, L., Roche, H. M., German, B. and van Ommen, B. (2005) Metabolomics in human nutrition: opportunities and challenges. The American journal of clinical nutrition. 82, 497-503

18   Gika, H. G., Theodoridis, G. A., Wingate, J. E. and Wilson, I. D. (2007) Within-day reproducibility of an HPLC-MS-based method for metabonomic analysis: application to human urine. Journal of proteome research. 6, 3291-3303

19   Gore, C. J., Parisotto, R., Ashenden, M. J., Stray-Gundersen, J., Sharpe, K., Hopkins, W., Emslie, K. R., Howe, C., Trout, G. J., Kazlauskas, R. and Hahn, A. G. (2003) Second-generation blood tests to detect erythropoietin abuse by athletes. Haematologica. 88, 333-344

20   Goto, K., Ishii, N., Sugihara, S., Yoshioka, T. and Takamatsu, K. (2007) Effects of resistance exercise on lipolysis during subsequent submaximal exercise. Medicine and science in sports and exercise. 39, 308-315

21   Grootveld, M. and Halliwell, B. (1987) Measurement of allantoin and uric acid in human body fluids. A potential index of free-radical reactions in vivo? The Biochemical journal. 243, 803-808

22   Hu, Q., Noll, R. J., Li, H., Makarov, A., Hardman, M. and Graham Cooks, R. (2005) The Orbitrap: a new mass spectrometer. J Mass Spectrom. 40, 430-443

23   Kamleh, M. A., Hobani, Y., Dow, J. A., Zheng, L. and Watson, D. G. (2009) Towards a platform for the metabonomic profiling of different strains of Drosophila melanogaster using liquid chromatography-Fourier transform mass spectrometry. The FEBS journal. 276, 6798-6809

24   Koal, T. and Deigner, H. P. Challenges in mass spectrometry based targeted metabolomics. Current molecular medicine. 10, 216-226

25   Lavoie, C., Diguet, A., Milot, M. and Gareau, R. (1998) Erythropoietin (rHuEPO) doping: effects of exercise on anaerobic metabolism in rats. International journal of sports medicine. 19, 281-286

26   Lewis, G. D., Farrell, L., Wood, M. J., Martinovic, M., Arany, Z., Rowe, G. C., Souza, A., Cheng, S., McCabe, E. L., Yang, E., Shi, X., Deo, R., Roth, F. P., Asnani, A., Rhee, E. P., Systrom, D. M., Semigran, M. J., Vasan, R. S., Carr, S. A., Wang, T. J., Sabatine, M. S., Clish, C. B. and Gerszten, R. E. Metabolic signatures of exercise in human plasma. Science translational medicine. 2, 33ra37

27   Lewis, G. D., Wei, R., Liu, E., Yang, E., Shi, X., Martinovic, M., Farrell, L., Asnani, A., Cyrille, M., Ramanathan, A., Shaham, O., Berriz, G., Lowry, P. A., Palacios, I. F., Tasan, M., Roth, F. P., Min, J., Baumgartner, C., Keshishian, H., Addona, T., Mootha, V. K., Rosenzweig, A., Carr, S. A., Fifer, M. A., Sabatine, M. S. and Gerszten, R. E. (2008) Metabolite profiling of blood from individuals undergoing planned myocardial infarction reveals early markers of myocardial injury. The Journal of clinical investigation. 118, 3503-3512

28   Lutz, U., Lutz, R. W. and Lutz, W. K. (2006) Metabolic profiling of glucuronides in human urine by LC-MS/MS and partial least-squares discriminant analysis for classification and prediction of gender. Analytical chemistry. 78, 4564-4571

29   Maher, A. D., Zirah, S. F., Holmes, E. and Nicholson, J. K. (2007) Experimental and analytical variation in human urine in 1H NMR spectroscopy-based metabolic phenotyping studies. Analytical chemistry. 79, 5204-5211

30   Makarov, A., Denisov, E., Lange, O. and Horning, S. (2006) Dynamic range of mass accuracy in LTQ Orbitrap hybrid mass spectrometer. Journal of the American Society for Mass Spectrometry. 17, 977-982

31   Manitius, J., Szolkiewicz, M., Mysliwska, J., Zorena, K., Mysliwski, A., Jakubowski, Z., Lysiak-Szydlowska, W. and Rutkowski, B. (1995) Influence of 'nonhematological' doses of erythropoietin on lipid-carbohydrate metabolism and life quality in hemodialysis patients. Nephron. 69, 363-364

32   Meierhenrich, R., Jedicke, H., Voigt, A. and Lange, H. (1996) The effect of erythropoietin on lactate, pyruvate and excess lactate under physical exercise in dialysis patients. Clinical nephrology. 45, 90-97

33   Michlmayr, A., Oehler, R. (2010) 'OMICS': state of the art *in vitro* techniques employed in surgical research. Eur Surg. 42/3: 127-133

34   Mitchell, S., Holmes, E. and Carmichael, P. (2002) Metabonomics and medicine: the Biochemical Oracle. Biologist (London, England). 49, 217-221

35   Parisotto, R., Gore, C. J., Emslie, K. R., Ashenden, M. J., Brugnara, C., Howe, C., Martin, D. T., Trout, G. J. and Hahn, A. G. (2000) A novel method utilising markers of

altered erythropoiesis for the detection of recombinant human erythropoietin abuse in athletes. Haematologica. 85, 564-572

36   Pociot, F., Reimers, J. I. and Andersen, H. U. (1993) Nicotinamide--biological actions and therapeutic potential in diabetes prevention. IDIG Workshop, Copenhagen, Denmark, 4-5 December 1992. Diabetologia. 36, 574-576

37   Robach, P., Calbet, J. A., Thomsen, J. J., Boushel, R., Mollard, P., Rasmussen, P. and Lundby, C. (2008) The ergogenic effect of recombinant human erythropoietin on VO2max depends on the severity of arterial hypoxemia. PloS one. 3, e2996

38   Rochfort, S. (2005) Metabolomics reviewed: a new "omics" platform technology for systems biology and implications for natural products research. Journal of natural products. 68, 1813-1820

39   Scalbert, A., Brennan, L., Fiehn, O., Hankemeier, T., Kristal, B. S., van Ommen, B., Pujos-Guillot, E., Verheij, E., Wishart, D. and Wopereis, S. (2009) Mass-spectrometry-based metabolomics: limitations and recommendations for future progress with particular focus on nutrition research. Metabolomics. 5, 435-458

40   Scheltema, R. A., Kamleh, A., Wildridge, D., Ebikeme, C., Watson, D. G., Barrett, M. P., Jansen, R. C. and Breitling, R. (2008) Increasing the mass accuracy of high-resolution LC-MS data using background ions: a case study on the LTQ-Orbitrap. Proteomics. 8, 4647-4656

41   Shaham, O., Wei, R., Wang, T. J., Ricciardi, C., Lewis, G. D., Vasan, R. S., Carr, S. A., Thadhani, R., Gerszten, R. E. and Mootha, V. K. (2008) Metabolic profiling of the human response to a glucose challenge reveals distinct axes of insulin sensitivity. Molecular systems biology. 4, 214

42   Ulrich, E. L., Akutsu, H., Doreleijers, J. F., Harano, Y., Ioannidis, Y. E., Lin, J., Livny, M., Mading, S., Maziuk, D., Miller, Z., Nakatani, E., Schulte, C. F., Tolmie, D. E., Kent Wenger, R., Yao, H. and Markley, J. L. (2008) BioMagResBank. Nucleic acids research. 36, D402-408

43   Varlet-Marie, E., Audran, M., Lejeune, M., Bonafoux, B., Sicart, M. T., Marti, J., Piquemal, D. and Commes, T. (2004) Analysis of human reticulocyte genes reveals altered erythropoiesis: potential use to detect recombinant human erythropoietin doping. Haematologica. 89, 991-997

44   Walsh, M. C., Brennan, L., Malthouse, J. P., Roche, H. M. and Gibney, M. J. (2006) Effect of acute dietary standardization on the urinary, plasma, and salivary metabolomic profiles of healthy humans. The American journal of clinical nutrition. 84, 531-539

45   Want, E. J., Nordstrom, A., Morita, H. and Siuzdak, G. (2007) From exogenous to endogenous: the inevitable imprint of mass spectrometry in metabolomics. Journal of proteome research. 6, 459-468

46   Watson, D. G. The potential of mass spectrometry for the global profiling of parasite metabolomes. Parasitology. 137, 1409-1423

47   Yan, B., A, J., Wang, G., Lu, H., Huang, X., Liu, Y., Zha, W., Hao, H., Zhang, Y., Liu, L., Gu, S., Huang, Q., Zheng, Y. and Sun, J. (2009) Metabolomic investigation into variation of endogenous metabolites in professional athletes subject to strength-endurance training. J Appl Physiol. 106, 531-538